DR.GRACE

HESTER

.Dr. Grace Hester stands at the intersection of health, passion, and culinary excellence. A distinguished medical professional and accomplished nutritionist, she seamlessly weaves together her expertise to create a holistic approach to well-being.

Dr. Hester earned her medical degree from the renowned Johns Hopkins School of Medicine, consistently ranked among the top medical schools globally. Her commitment to advancing healthcare led her to prestigious positions at the Mayo Clinic, where she honed her skills in internal medicine. Driven by a desire to explore the profound connection between nutrition and overall health, she furthered her education at the Culinary Institute of America.

– With a deep understanding of both medicine and nutrition, Dr. Hester embarked on a mission to inspire others to embrace a healthier lifestyle. Her culinary journey– led to the creation of a series of cookbooks that blend the art of cooking with the scienc–e of nutrition. Each recipe is a testament to her commitment to flavor, nourishment, and well-being.

Currently, Dr. Hester serves as the Chief Nutritionist at the renowned Cleveland Clinic, where she continues to innovate in the field of nutritional medicine. Her groundbreaking work has been recognized not only within the medical community but also by a broader audience seeking practical and delicious ways to enhance their health.

B

 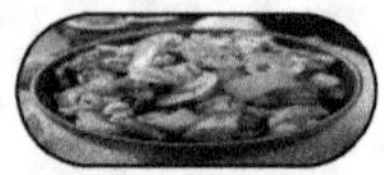

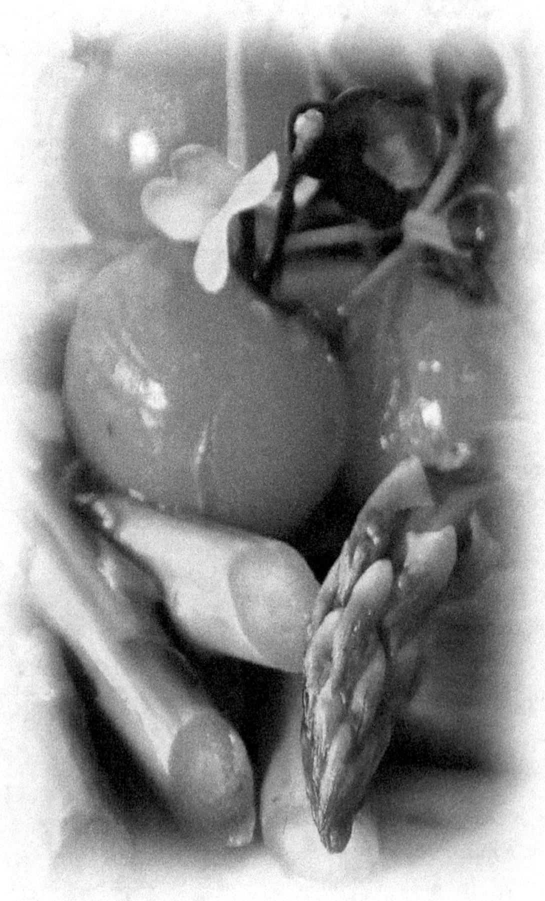

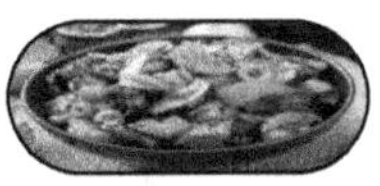

TABLE OF CONTENT

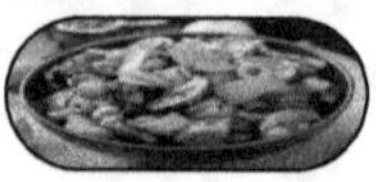

FERTILITY

COOKBOOK

FOR

COUPLES

My Secrete Delicious Recipes For Boasting Your Chances of Getting Pregnant.

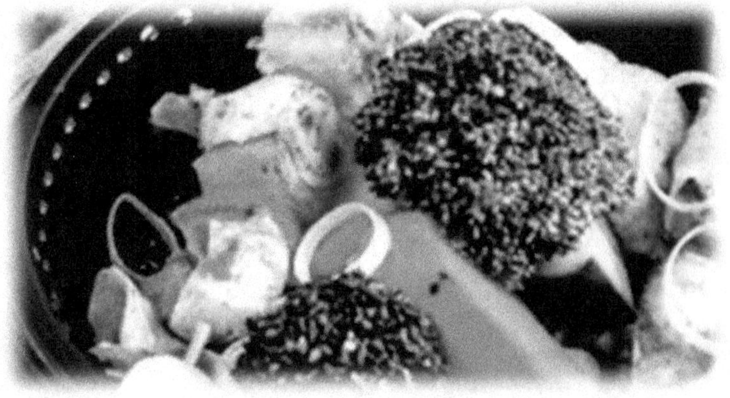

Dr. Grace Hester A.kaboo Publishing —

 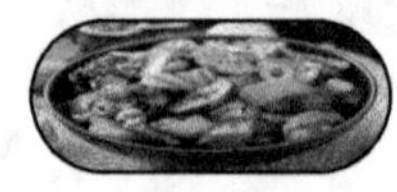

Copyright Page]

Copyright ©2023] by Dr.Grace Hester

—Disclaimer: The recipes contained in this cookbook are intended for personal use and enjoyment. The author and publisher are not responsible for any health issues or allergic reactions that may arise from the use of the ingredients or recipes provided. It is recommended that individuals with specific dietary concerns or restrictions consult a qualified healthcare professional.

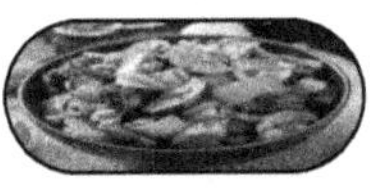

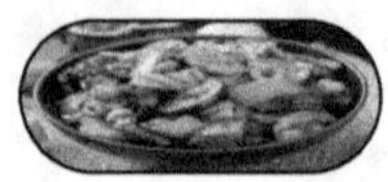

INTRODUCTION

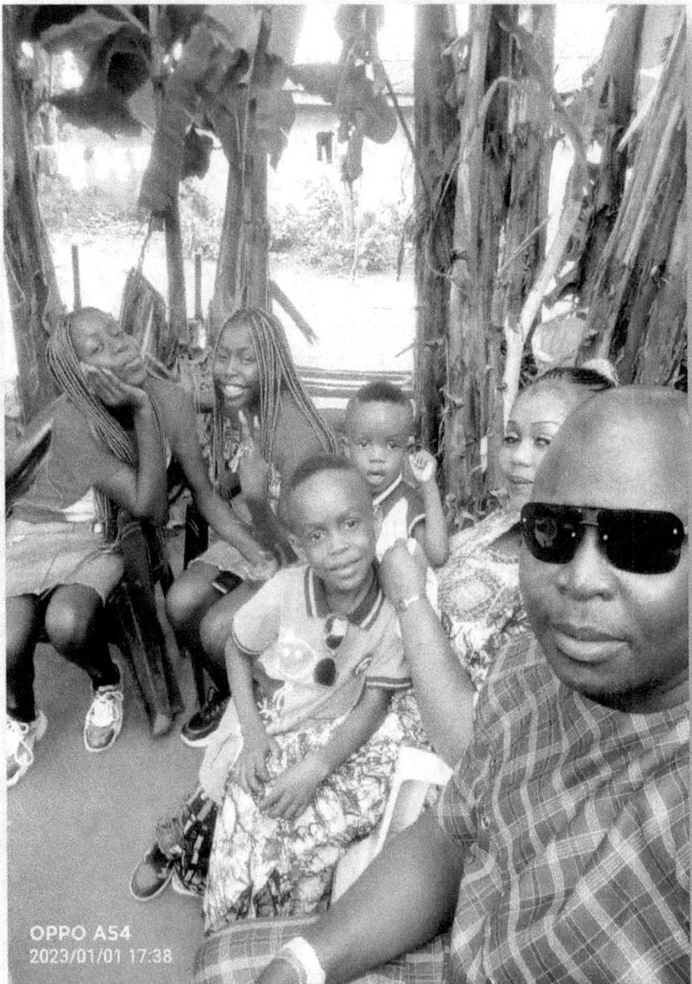

 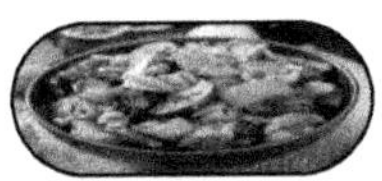

TRUE LIFE TESTIMONY

The five-year journey that Mr. and Mrs. Emeka took to become parents was profound and heartbreaking. They were a passionately in love couple with dreams of starting a family who were from the stunning sceneries of Nigeria. But infertility was a harsh twist that fate had in store for them.

Their tale starts in a sleepy village where children's laughter and footsteps filled the air. However, this song of life eluded the Emeka family. With each passing day, their desire for a child became stronger, and numerous trips to the doctor's office only made their need worse.

Mrs. Emeka found a ray of hope one fateful afternoon when the sun showered the community in its golden radiance. Mrs. Adewale, a neighbor, had been relating tales of her own struggles with infertility. She mentioned "The Fertility Diet Cookbook" by Hester, a fascinating book that she had recently discovered. Mrs. Emeka was intrigued and made the decision to look for this culinary gem in the hopes that it would change their life.

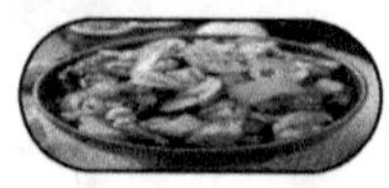

Mr. and Mrs. Emeka bought the cookbook and plunged into its pages with unyielding determination. The recipes in the book weren't just regular dishes; rather, they were a carefully curated variety made to increase fertility organically. The recipe book was a gold mine of information, brimming with ingredients and culinary methods that carried the promise of a better tomorrow.

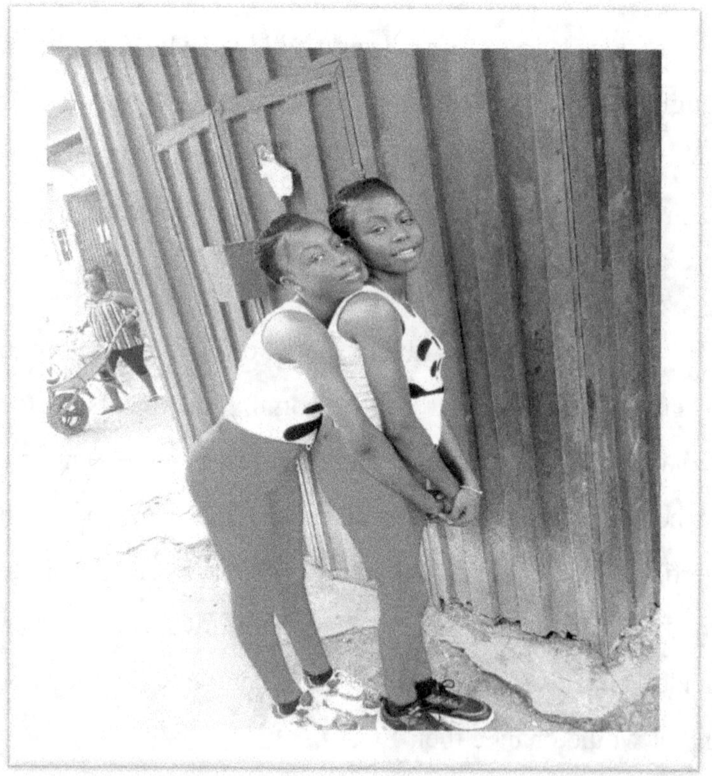

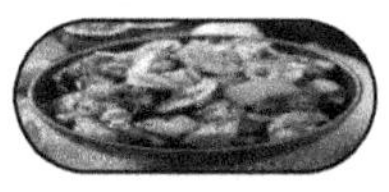

The Emekas adopted the recipes one at a time, weighing each ingredient precisely and cooking with love and devotion. Each meal seem–s to embody the core of their dreams. Their kitchen was filled with the aroma of fresh herbs, the sizzle of the pan, and the scent of spices, which inspired optimism and anticipation.

There were obstacles along the way. The Emekas had their doubts about their decision to adhere to the diet strictly at times. But as they endured the ups and downs of their struggle with infertility, they held hands and reminded each other of their shared dream.

As the weeks stretched into months, a subtle change started to happen inside of their bodies. Mrs. Emeka noted a rise in her energy levels, a radiance to her skin, and an improvement in her general wellbeing. Mr. Emeka also felt a renewed vigor for the first time in years.

A thunderclap that reverberated throughout the town on a rainy night marked the turning point in their narrative and roused them from their slumber. Mrs. Emeka had been meticulously monitoring her ovulation cycle, and that particular night, everything seemed to come together. Their

 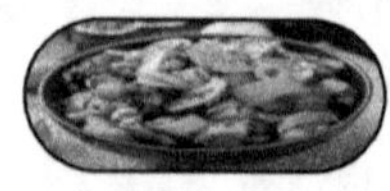

love grew into a deed that would alter both of their lives forever in a moment of ferocious passion and need.

Months went by while anticipation lingered in the air like a light breeze. The Emekas remained steadfast in their resolve to cooking the recipes from the cookbook that would increase fertility. In anticipation of the news they had been waiting to hear, they held hands while seeing the doctor.

Then, on this lovely morning, the doctor's comments caused them to cry with happiness. Mrs. Emeka had a baby! The voyage that had started with the turning of a page in a cookbook had arrived.

The Emekas' happiness grew as the months passed. They started to think about the lives they would create for their soon-to-arrive children as their parental fantasies became more real. They decorated the room, placed toys inside, and sang lullabies to the baby all night long.

Mrs. Emeka went into labor on a day when the sun bathed the sky in hues of orange and pink. The sound of her focused breathing and Mr. Emeka's unflinching support

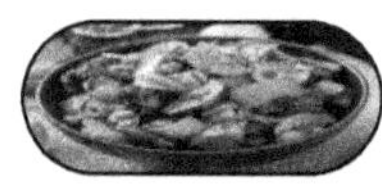

Reverberated throughout the hospital room. Victory and Favour, their twins, were born, and their screams signaled the beginning of a new chapter in the Emeka family's history.

The twins' birth was nothing short of a miracle, demonstrating the strength of love, willpower, and the extraordinary effects of the fertility diet. Mr. and Mrs. Emeka realized that their journey had been worth every difficult minute and every tear they had shed as they held their beloved children in their arms.

Their tale immediately traveled throughout the community, giving hope to many who were struggling with infertility. The Emekas demonstrated that there was a way to success, and it started with the pages of "The Fertility Diet Cookbook" by Hester, shattering the shame and silence surrounding the problem.

Victory and Favour offered their parents and the entire neighborhood a great deal of joy in the years that followed. Their laughter reverberated throughout the entire hamlet, serving as a poignant reminder that even the most difficult obstacles could be conquered with unshakeable resolve and the proper formula for success.

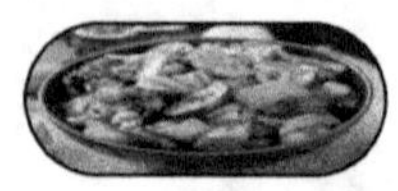

The Emekas' story of success acted as a light of hope for others seeking to have families of their own. The Emekas understood that their voyage had not only given them a family but also sparked a flame of hope that would continue to burn brilliantly for subsequent generations as the sun sank over the hamlet, producing a warm and reassuring glow.

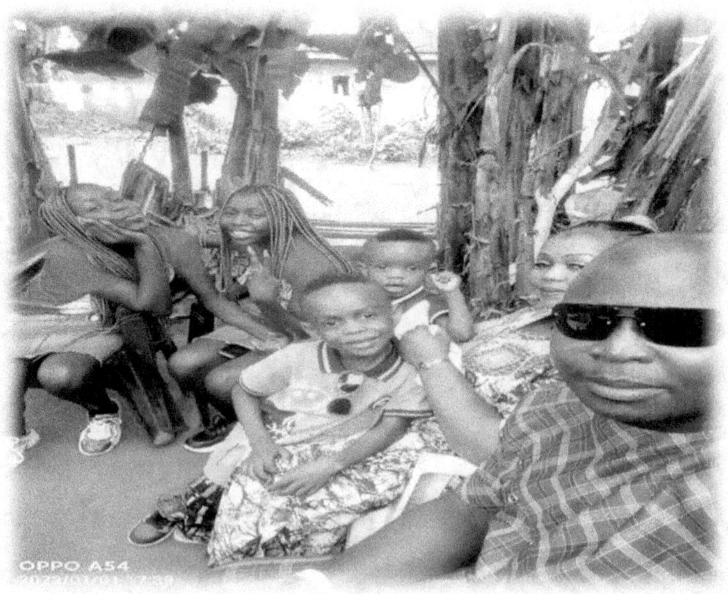

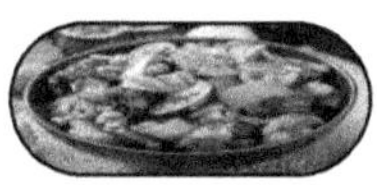

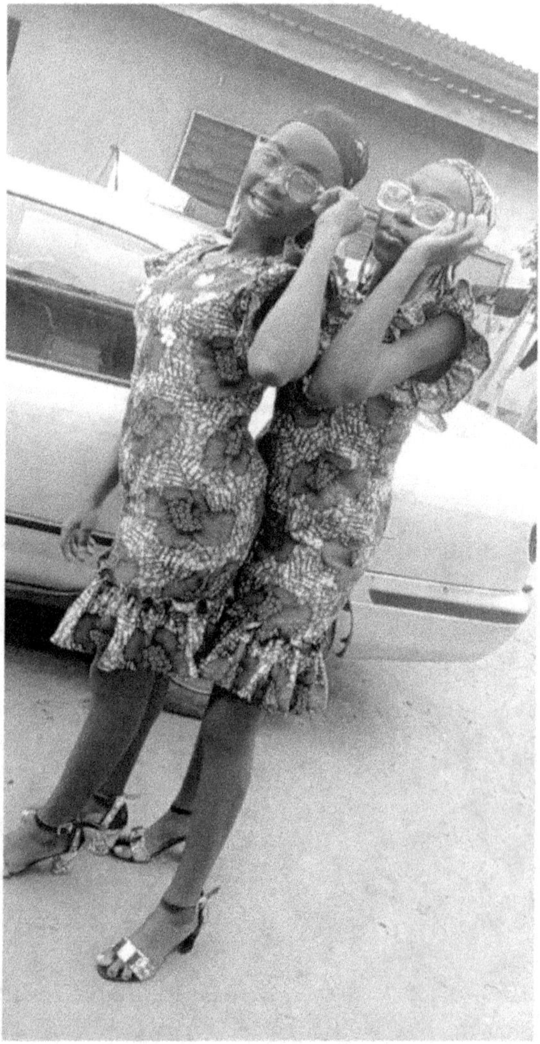

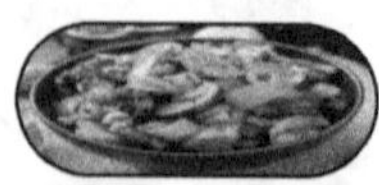

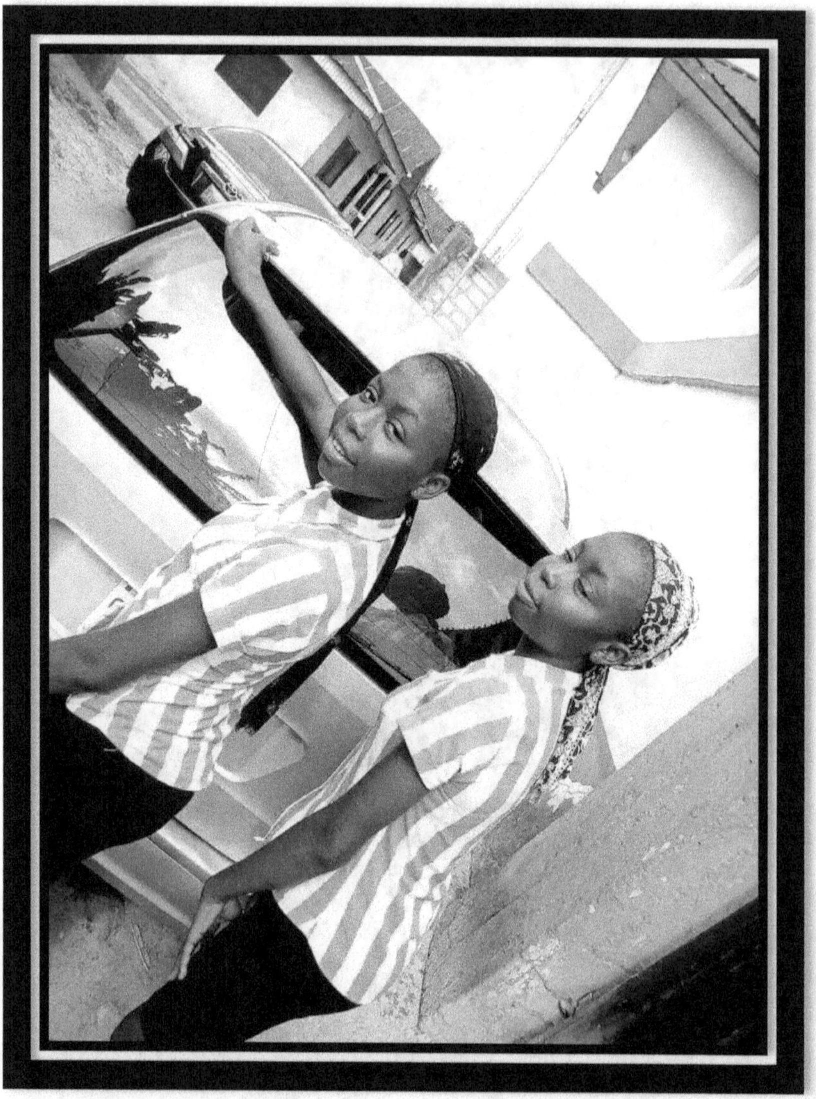

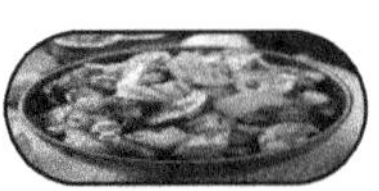

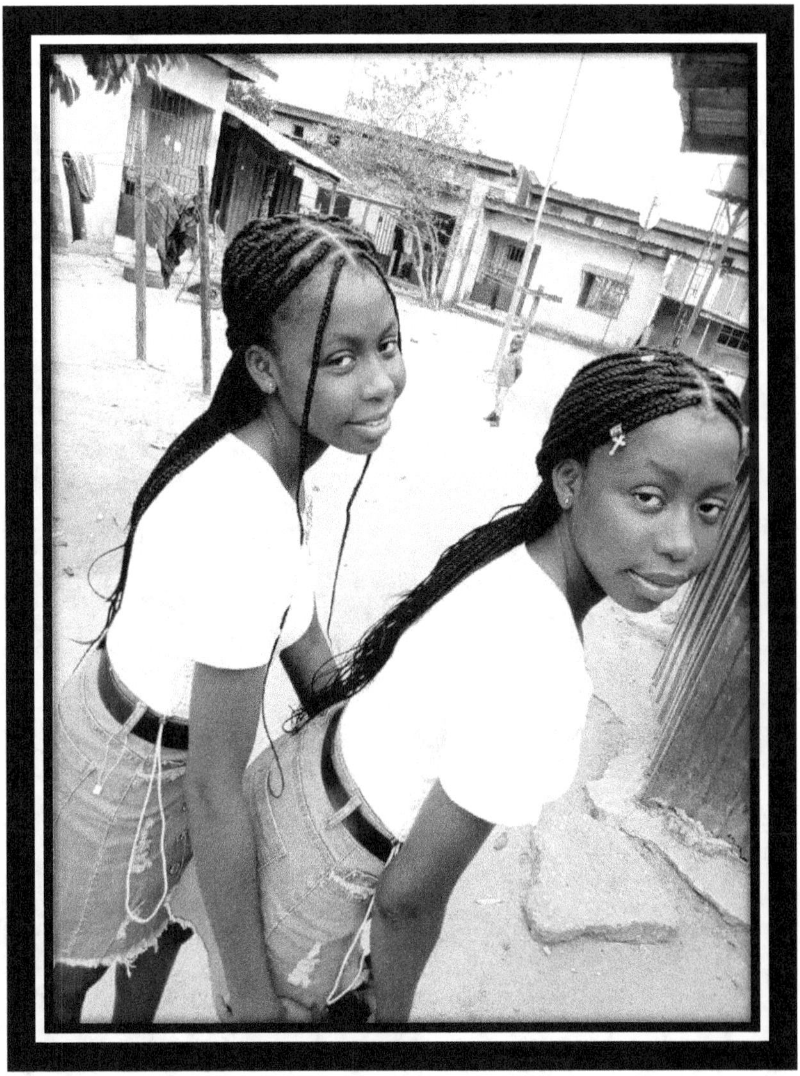

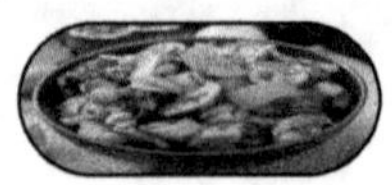

Nutrition for fertility

Getting Enough Protein Can Improve Your Fertility

Proteins are essential for life and have a big impact on fertility. They help reproductive hormones like progesterone and estrogen grow and remain stable. Adequate protein intake can improve ovulation by regulating menstrual cycles. Lean meats, fish, eggs, and plant-based choices like beans and nuts are some sources of high-quality protein.

The Importance of Healthy Fats in Fats and Oils

Fertility depends on good fats, including the monounsaturated and polyunsaturated fats in fatty fish, avocados, and olive oil. These fats may help treat diseases like polycystic ovarian syndrome (PCOS) or endometriosis because they regulate hormone production and lower inflammation.

 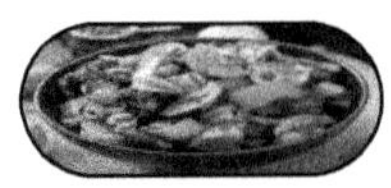

The Balance between Carbohydrates and Blood Sugar

Whole grains, fruits, and vegetables all include complex carbs that give you a continuous amount of energy and help keep your blood sugar levels under control. Infertility might result from hormonal imbalance caused by high blood sugar. An adequate level of fertility can be supported by a balanced carbohydrate consumption.

Minerals and Vitamins:

Micronutrients Are Important

Folate:

Folic acid, which is present in leafy greens and meals that have been fortified, is essential for early embryonic development and may help to prevent birth abnormalities.

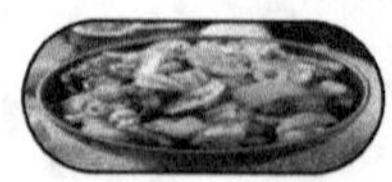

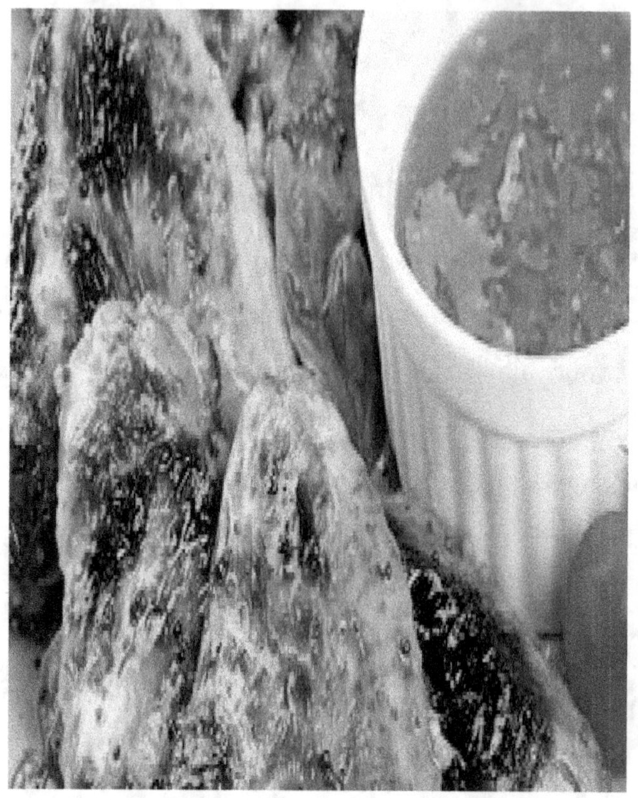

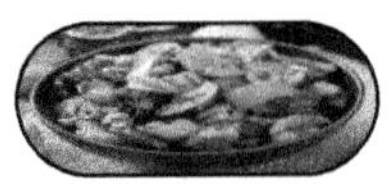

Iron:

Foods high in iron, such as spinach and lean red meat, can avoid anemia, which can impair fertility.

Zinc:

This mineral is prevalent in seafood and nuts and is important for the health of eggs and the generation of hormones.

Vitamin D:

This vitamin, which is linked to better fertility and reproductive health, can be obtained from the sun and fortified foods.

Salmon and other fatty fish include omega-3 fatty acids, which maintain hormone balance and prevent inflammation.

Safeguarding the health of sperm and eggs

Fruits and vegetables that are high in antioxidants like vitamin C and E aid to prevent oxidative damage to eggs and sperm, increasing overall fertility.

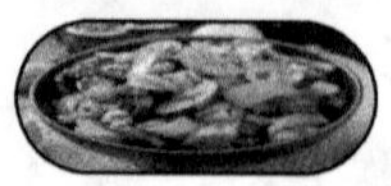

Fiber:

Gut Well-Being and Hormone Harmony

Fiber from vegetables, fruits, and whole grains facilitates digestion and encourages hormonal balance. Fertility can benefit from improved food absorption caused by a healthy gut.

Water:

Drinking Water Is Important for Reproductive Health

Although sometimes disregarded, adequate hydration is essential for general health, including reproductive health. Water promotes biological processes and aids in the transportation of nutrients.

Hydration:

An Underrated Hero

The best conditions for conception are created by maintaining appropriate hydration, which supports all of the body's processes, including hormone balance.

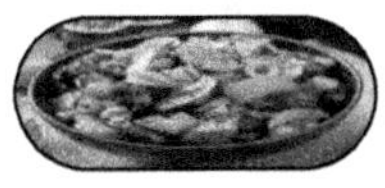

To sum up, a diet with an emphasis on promoting fertility that is high in protein, healthy fats, complex carbs, vitamins, minerals, antioxidants, fiber, and water can significantly improve reproductive health. These nutrients may be able to reverse the causes of infertility and increase the likelihood of conception through regulating hormones, reducing inflammation, and supporting general health. Keep in mind that a customized fertility diet plan requires consultation with a medical practitioner or nutritionist.

Numerous factors can contribute to infertility, which affects millions of couples worldwide and is extremely distressing. In this post, we'll look at some of the main causes of infertility and consider some dietary modifications and meals that might be able to help it get better.

CAUSES OF INFERTILITY

OVULATORY DISORDERS: For women, infertility is frequently brought on by irregular or absent ovulation. The hormonal balance is disturbed by conditions like Polycystic

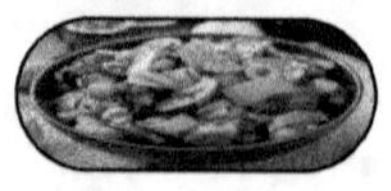

Ovary Syndrome (PCOS), which prevents the regular release of eggs.

SPERM HEALTH: Low sperm counts or poor sperm quality are frequent causes of male infertility. Smoking, binge drinking, and obesity are some examples of factors that can impair sperm function and production.

Issues with the fallopian tubes can prevent the fertilized egg from making it to the uterus, which can result in infertility. This issue may be exacerbated by infections, pelvic inflammatory disease, or endometriosis.

AGE:

Because of a drop in the quantity and quality of eggs, women's fertility naturally diminishes as they age. This makes conception more difficult, especially for women over the age of 35.

LIFESTYLE FACTORS:

Both men and women might have reduced fertility as a result of unhealthy lifestyle choices such as excessive stress, obesity, and smoking. While obesity can cause

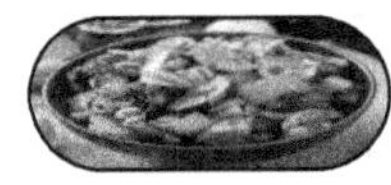

hormonal abnormalities and insulin resistance, stress can disturb hormonal balance.

CHRONIC ILLNESSES:

By interfering with hormone balance, many medical ailments like diabetes, thyroid problems, and autoimmune diseases can affect fertility.

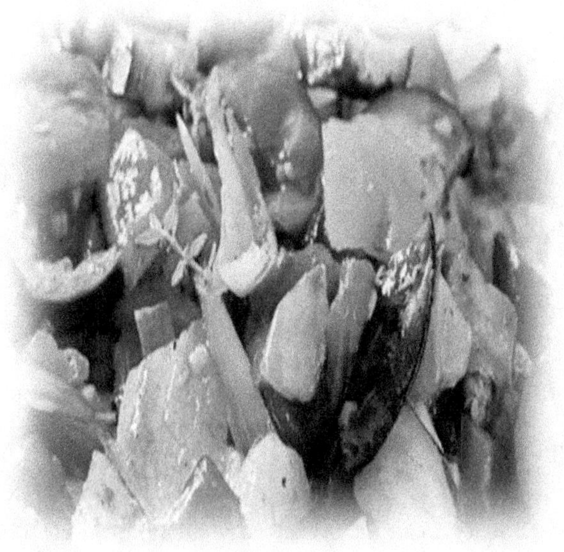

—

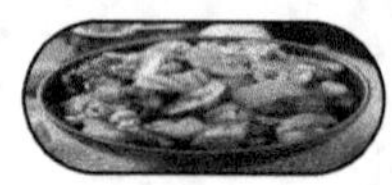

Meals and Diet as a
Potential Fix:

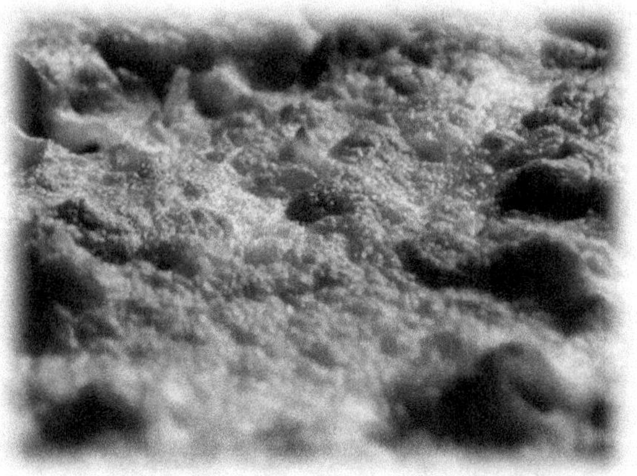

In order to address some of the causes of infertility and enhance overall reproductive health, dietary changes might be quite important. This is how:

Hormone regulation can be aided by eating a diet that is well-balanced and full of fresh produce, whole grains, lean meats, and healthy fats. For instance, meals high in omega-3 fatty acids, such as salmon and flaxseeds, may enhance the caliber of eggs and the health of sperm.–

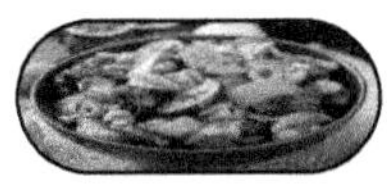

CONTROLLING WEIGHT:

Fertility depends on maintaining a healthy weight. Extra body fat can cause insulin resistance, which interferes with the production of hormones. A healthy diet and consistent exercise can help you manage your weight.

REDUCING INFLAMMATION:

Infertility problems may be exacerbated by chronic inflammation. Berry and leafy greens are two examples of foods high in antioxidants that can help reduce inflammation and support a healthier reproductive system.

Reproductive health can be safeguarded by avoiding or reducing exposure to environmental toxins, such as those in some processed foods, pesticides, and pollution. It can be advantageous to choose organic vegetables and stay away from processed foods.

FOLIC ACID:

Folic acid is essential for preventing birth abnormalities and maintaining a healthy pregnancy and is present in leafy greens and fortified cereals. It should be a part of both partners' diets.–

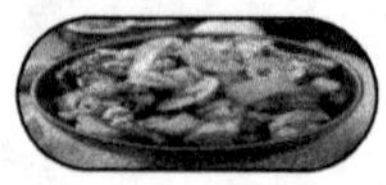

LIMITING ALCOHOL AND CAFFEINE:

Drinking too much alcohol or caffeine can be harmful to fertility. Couples who are trying to get pregnant may find it helpful to cut back on these substances.

STRESS MANAGEMENT:

Stress management practices like yoga, meditation, and mindfulness can be incorporated into everyday routines to assist manage stress, which may then enhance fertility.

It's crucial to remember that while making dietary adjustments can be a good first step in resolving infertility, they may not always be the best course of action. Infertile couples should seek the advice of medical professionals, such as reproductive endocrinologists, to determine the precise causes and potential solutions that might work best for them.

In conclusion, a range of factors, including hormonal imbalances, lifestyle decisions, and aging-related changes, might contribute to infertility. While meals and a healthy diet might be helpful in resolving some of these problems, fertility treatment should take a holistic approach.

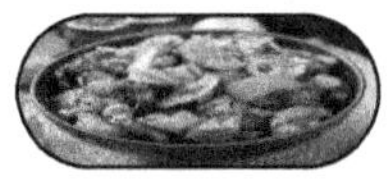

To decide the best course of action for each couple's particular circumstances, it is crucial to seek medical counsel and guidance.

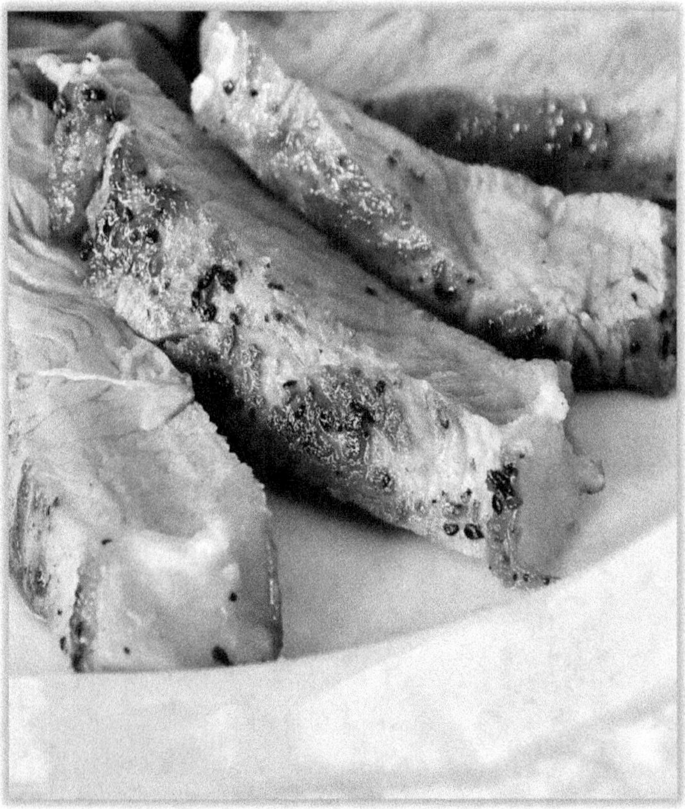

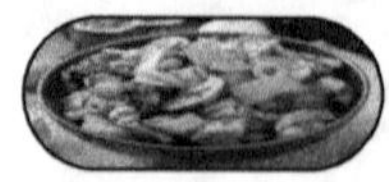

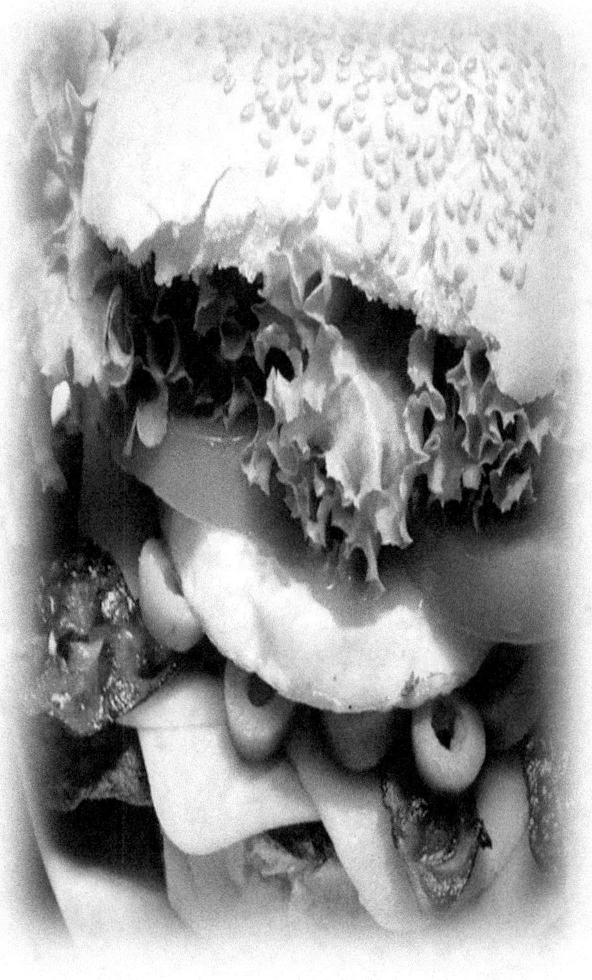

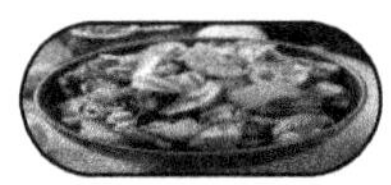

Breakfast Fertility Recipes

A parfait of Greek yogurt

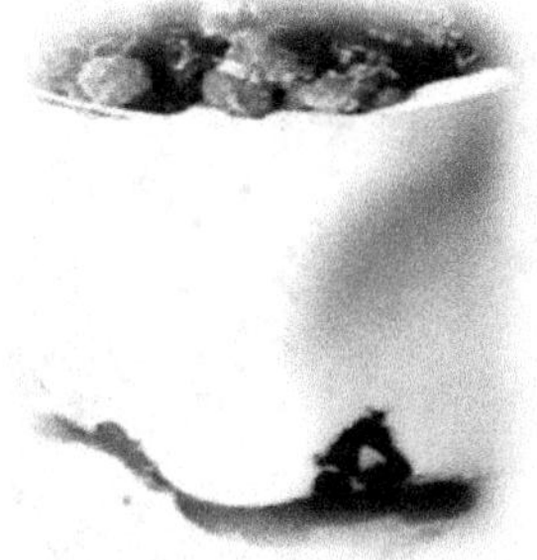

INGREDIENTS:

- Greek yogurt, one cup
- Berry mixture of blueberries, strawberries, and raspberries, 1/2 cup
- Honey, two tablespoons–

 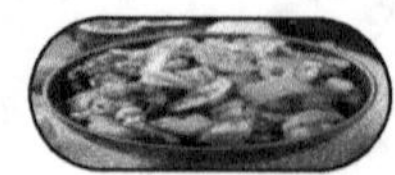

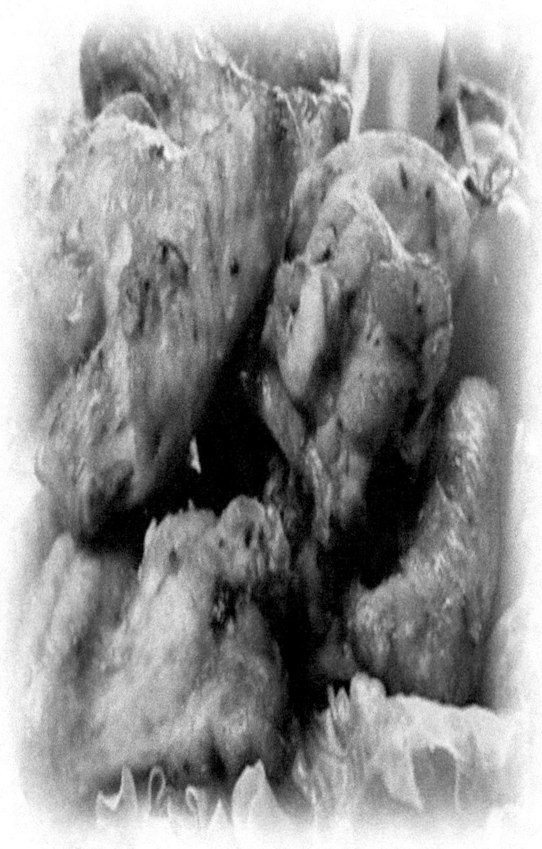 1/4 cup of cereal

 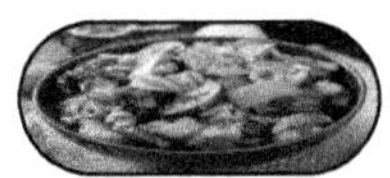

NUTRITIVE WORTH:

- 15g of protein
- 4g of fiber

Preparation Time: 5 minutes

PREPARATION:

Preparation Greek yogurt, mixed berries, honey, and granola are layered in a bowl.

Serve right away.

Omelet with spinach and mushrooms

INGREDIENTS:

- two eggs, big
- 4 ounces of chopped spinach
- Sliced mushrooms in 1/4 cup
- Parmesan cheese, grated, in 2 tablespoons
- pepper and salt as desired

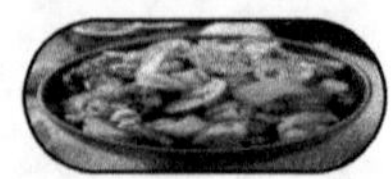

NUTRITIVE WORTH:

- 14g of protein
- 2g of fiber

10 minutes for cooking

PREPARATION

In a bowl, ensure you properly turn or stir together the eggs likewise salt, and pepper.

In a pan, cook spinach and mushrooms until they are tender.

Cheese should be sprinkled on top of the eggs before they are cooked till set.

Breakfast bowl with quinoa

INGREDIENTS:

- half a cup of cooked quinoa.
- 14 cup of almond slices
- 14 cup of peaches, diced
- 1 teaspoon of honey—

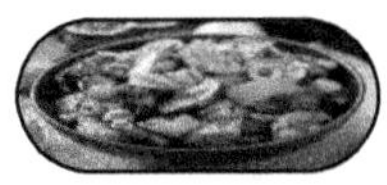

NUTRITIVE WORTH:

❖ 7g protein

❖ 5g of fiber

15 minutes (for quinoa preparation)

The ingredients for this dish include quinoa, almonds, peaches, and honey.

Mix thoroughly, then indulge.

Poached eggs on avocado toast

INGREDIENTS:

- 1 ripe avocado and two pieces of whole-grain bread
- two huge eggs
- pepper and salt as desired

NUTRITIVE WORTH:

- 13g of protein
- 6g of fiber

—

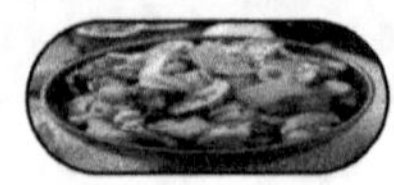

15 minutes for cooking

PREPARATION

- Toasting bread is a method of preparation.
- On the toast, mash the avocado.
- Add poached eggs to the top.
- Add salt and pepper to taste.

Berry Smoothie

INGREDIENTS:

- One cup of mixed berries with strawberries, blueberries, and raspberries within
- Greek yogurt, half a cup
- 50 ml of almond milk
- a tsp. of flaxseeds
- 1 teaspoon of honey
- nutritive worth:
- 10g of protein
- 6g of fiber

Preparation Time: 5 minutes–

Blend each item until it is smooth to prepare.

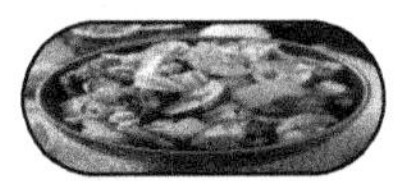

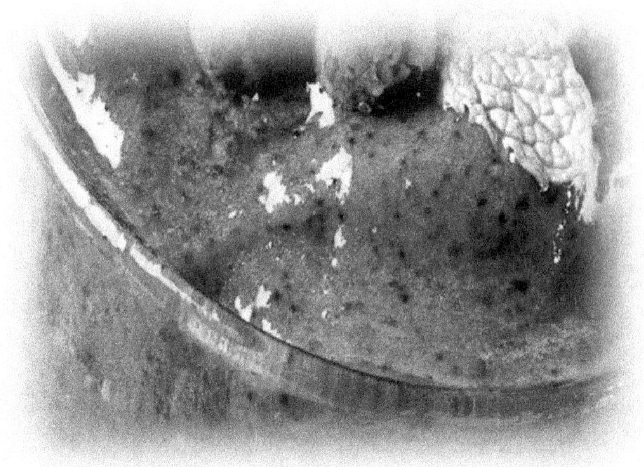

Sweet Potato Hash

INGREDIENTS:

- 1 chopped sweet potato
- 12 chopped onion
- 1 diced bell pepper
- 2 eggs
- Olive oil, 1 tbsp

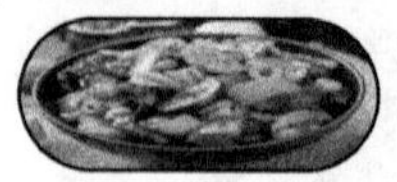

NUTRITIVE WORTH:

- ❖ 9g protein
- ❖ 5g of fiber

20 minutes for cooking

METHOD OF PREPARATION: Saute bell pepper, onion, and sweet potato in olive oil until soft.

Over the mixture, crack eggs, cover, and cook until the eggs are set.

Chia Seed Dessert

INGREDIENTS:

- Chia seeds, 2 tablespoons
- almond milk, 1 cup
- One-half teaspoon of vanilla extract
- maple syrup, 1 tbsp

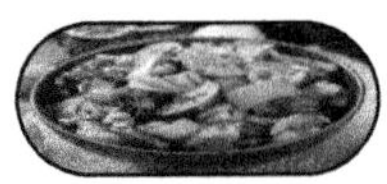

NUTRITIVE WORTH:

- 4g. protein
- 10g of fiber

5 minutes of cooking time + cooling

Chia seeds, almond milk, vanilla essence, and maple syrup should all be combined during preparation.

Stirring occasionally, chill for at least two hours.

Whole-grain pancakes

INGREDIENTS:

- whole wheat flour, 1 cup
- 1 teaspoon of honey
- one tablespoon of baking powder
- half a teaspoon of cinnamon
- almond milk, 1 cup

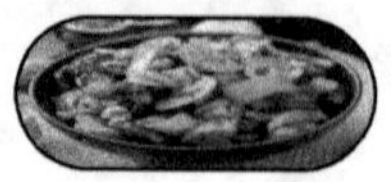

NUTRITIVE WORTH:

- 6g protein
- 4g of fiber

15 minutes for cooking

CREATING A PREPARATION:

Add the cinnamon, baking powder, honey, and flour together.

Add the almond milk and blend well.

On a griddle, cook pancakes till golden brown.

Toast with almond butter and banana

INGREDIENTS:

- Contains two pieces of whole-grain bread.
- Almond butter, two tablespoons
- Sliced banana, one

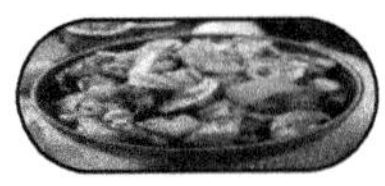

FOOD VALUE:

- ❖ 8g of protein
- ❖ 6g of fiber

Preparation Time: 5 minutes

Toast the toast, slather it with almond butter, and then top it with banana slices.

Vegetable breakfast burrito -

- 2 whole-grain tortillas -
- 2 scrambled eggs
- One-fourth cup black beans
- 1/4 cup tomatoes, diced
- 1/4 cup bell peppers, diced
- 2 teaspoons of salsa

- NUTRIENT CONTENT:

- 14g protein
- 6g fiber

- 15 minutes for cooking–

- Fill tortillas with eggs, black beans, tomatoes, and bell peppers.

 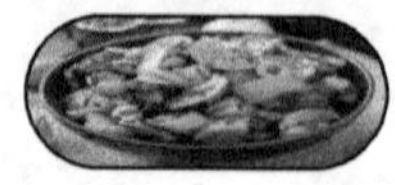

    ＋ Add salsa on top, fold, and eat.

42 | P a g e

These dishes include a variety of nutrients and can be included in a diet plan for conception. Adapt the amounts to your tastes and dietary requirements. Have a delicious and healthy breakfast!

—

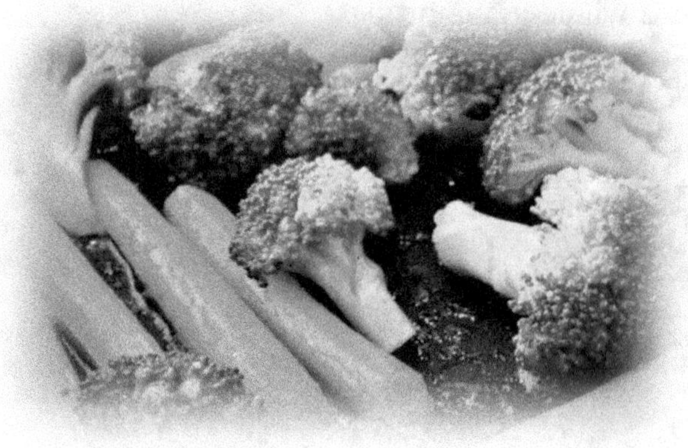

—

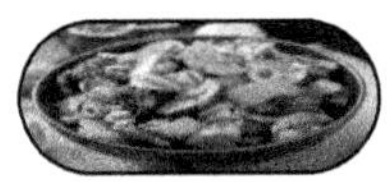

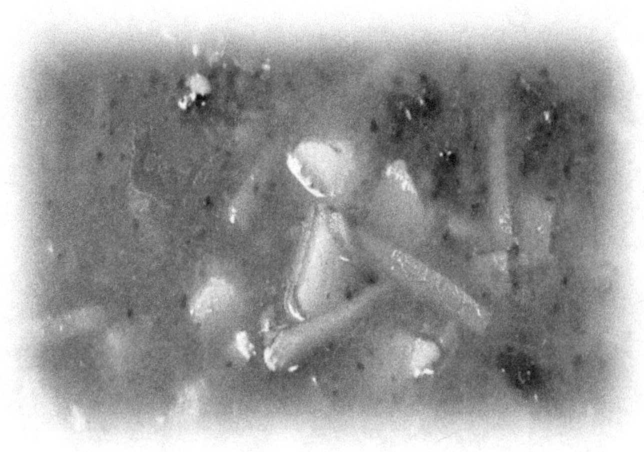

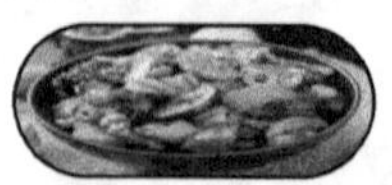

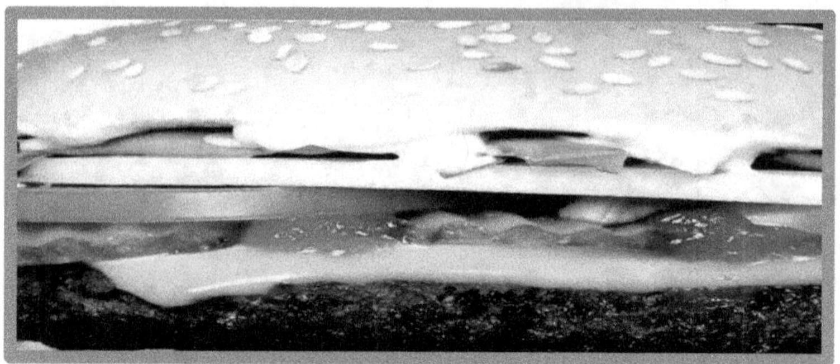

SALADS AND SOUPS

Soups that promote fertility

INGREDIENTS FOR SPINACH AND LENTIL SOUP:

- Dried green lentils, 1 cup
- 2 cups of fresh spinach leaves to 4 cups of vegetable broth
- 1 chopped onion, 2 minced garlic cloves, 1 chopped carrot, 1 chopped celery stalk, and 1 teaspoon of olive oil
- pepper and salt as desired

Iron, folate, and fiber content are all high.

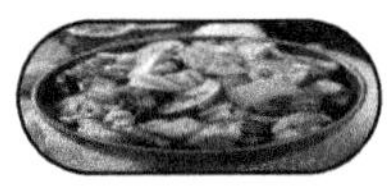

Time spent cooking: about 30 minutes.

Quinoa and tomato soup

COMPONENTS:

- 4 cups low-sodium tomato juice with 1 cup washed quinoa
- 1 chopped onion, 2 minced garlic cloves
- 1 chopped red bell pepper
- 1 teaspoon olive oil
- 1-teaspoon dried basil
- pepper and salt as desired

Rich in vitamins, proteins, and antioxidants, nutrition value.

Preparation Time: About 25 minutes.–

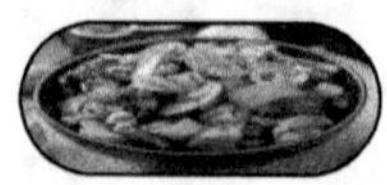

Broccoli and almond soup

INGREDIENTS

- 200 grams of broccoli florets
- 0.5 cup soaked and peeled almonds
- 1 diced onion, 2 minced garlic cloves
- 4 cups of veggie broth
- 1 teaspoon olive oil
- pepper and salt as desired

NUTRITIONAL VALUE: Rich in fiber, healthy fats, and vitamin E.

Time spent cooking: about 20 minutes.

Sweet Potato and Ginger Soup:

INGREDIENTS

- 2 big, peeled, and chopped sweet potatoes
- 1 onion, diced, 1 inch of fresh ginger, grated, and 4 cups of vegetable broth–

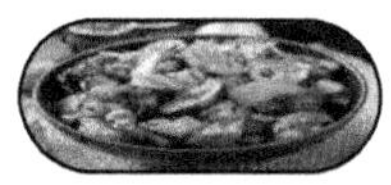

- 1 teaspoon olive oil
- pepper and salt as desired
- High in vitamin C and beta-carotene, with good nutritional value.

Preparation Time: About 30 minutes.

mushroom and barley soup:

INGREDIENTS FOR MUSHROOM AND BARLEY SOUP:

- one cup of pearl barley
- Sliced mushrooms, 8 ounces
- 1 diced onion, 2 minced garlic cloves
- 4 cups of veggie broth
- 1 teaspoon olive oil
- pepper and salt as desired

Rich in fiber, selenium, and B vitamins. High in nutritional value.

Time required for cooking: about 40 minutes.–

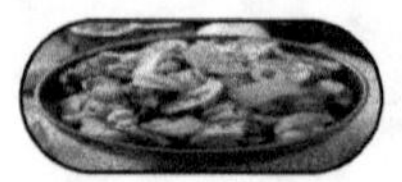

Salads that promote conception

Kale and Quinoa

KALE AND QUINOA SALAD INGREDIENTS:

- 1 cup of cooked and cooled quinoa
- 2 cups of chopped kale
- Pomegranate seeds in a half-cup
- 14 cup crumbled feta cheese
- Olive oil, 1/4 cup
- 1.5 tbsp lemon juice
- pepper and salt as desired

High in iron, folate, and antioxidants; high nutritional value.

Time Required for Preparation: 15 minutes.

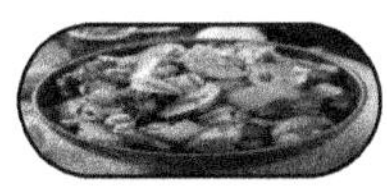

Beet and walnut salad:

INGREDIENTS FOR THE BEET AND WALNUT SALAD:

- 2 medium beets, cut after roasting
- 12 cup chopped walnuts
- 4 cups of greens, mixed
- Balsamic vinaigrette, 1/4 cup
- 1/4 cup crumbled goat cheese

Rich in folate, fiber, and omega-3 fatty acids; high in nutritional value.

30 minutes or so for preparation, including roasting the beets.

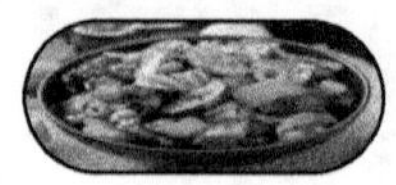

Avocado and Mango Salad:

INGREDIENTS FOR AVOCADO AND MANGO SALAD:

2 diced ripe avocados, 2 diced ripe mangoes, 1/2 finely chopped red onion, 1/4 cup chopped fresh cilantro, and 2 tablespoons lime juice

pepper and salt as desired

NUTRITIONAL VALUE:

Rich in vitamin C, folate, and good fats.

Time spent preparing: about 20 minutes.

spinach and berry salad:

INGREDIENTS

4 cups fresh leaves of spinach

1 cup of mixed berries, such as blueberries and strawberries

14 cup of almond slices

Balsamic vinaigrette, 2 tbsp

 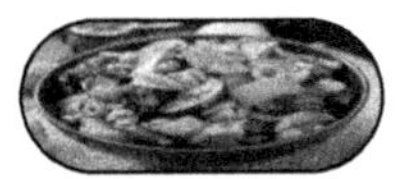

14 cup crumbled feta cheese

Iron, folate, and antioxidants are all abundant in this food.

Time spent preparing: about 15 minutes.

Chickpea and Cucumber Salad:

INGREDIENTS FOR CHICKPEA AND CUCUMBER SALAD:

- 2 cups washed and drained canned chickpeas
- cuke, one, diced
- 1 chopped red bell pepper
- 14 cup coarsely chopped red onion
- 2/TBS of olive oil
- 1.5 tbsp lemon juice
- pepper and salt as desired

Protein, fiber, and vitamin C levels are high.

Time Required for Preparation: 15 minutes.–

A number of nutrient-rich options for a fertility diet are offered by these recipes. Always remember to alter portion

 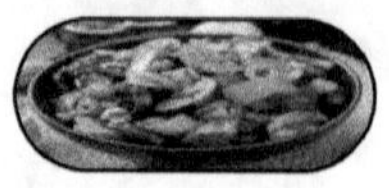

amounts and get specific advice from a healthcare professional.

Recipes For Vegetarians

Salad of spinach and chickpeas

INGREDIENTS:

- fresh spinach leaves in two cups
- 1 cup of rinsed and drained canned chickpeas
- Half a cup of cherry tomatoes
- Cucumber dice in a quarter cup
- Extra virgin olive oil, 2 tablespoons
- Lemon juice, 1 tablespoon
- Salt, 1/4 teaspoon
- Black pepper, 1/4 teaspoon

—

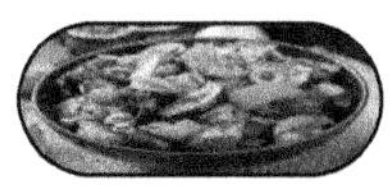

PREPARATION:

- Spinach, chickpeas, cherry tomatoes, and cucumber should all be combined in a big bowl.
- In a small bowl, whisk together the olive oil, lemon juice, salt, and pepper.
- Over the salad, drizzle the dressing, and give it a gentle stir.
- Serve right away.

VALUE NUTRITIVE (PER SERVING):

- 250 calories
- 8g protein
- 7g of fiber
- 120mcg Folate
- 3 mg. iron

15 minutes for cooking

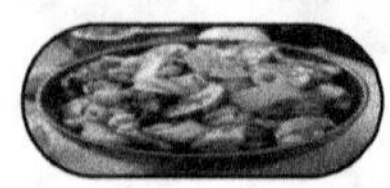

. Bowl of quinoa and black beans

INGREDIENTS:

quinoa boiled to 1 cup

- 1 cup of rinsed and drained canned black beans
- a half cup of colored bell peppers, chopped
- Red onion dice in a quarter cup
- 1/4 cup freshly chopped cilantro
- Lime juice, 2 tablespoons
- Olive oil, 1 tbsp
- Cumin, half a teaspoon
- pepper and salt as desired

PREPARATION:

- Cooked quinoa, black beans, bell peppers, red onion, and cilantro should all be combined in a big bowl.
- Combine lime juice, cumin, olive oil, salt, and pepper in a small bowl.
- Drizzle the dressing over the quinoa mixture and toss to combine.

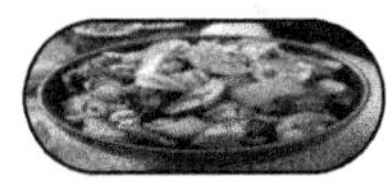

- cold or warm serving.

VALUE NUTRITIVE (PER SERVING):

- 320 calories
- 10g of protein
- 8g of fiber
- 100mcg Folate
- 2.5 mg. iron

Cooking Time: 20 minutes (if no pre-cooked quinoa is used)

Curry with sweet potatoes and lentils

INGREDIENTS:

- 2 cups of sweet potatoes, diced
- 1 cup of red lentils, dry
- one sliced onion
- 2 minced garlic cloves
- 14 oz. of diced tomatoes from a can
- Curry powder, two tablespoons–
- Turmeric, 1 teaspoon

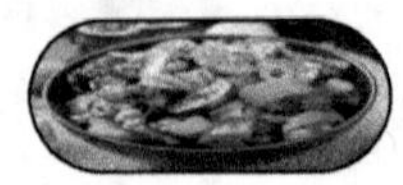

- Cumin, 1 teaspoon
- Chili powder, 1/2 teaspoon (adjust to taste)
- a mug of veggie broth and two
- pepper and salt as desired
- Olive oil, 2 tablespoons

PREPARATION:

in a big pot the olive oil should be heated in an average heat. Sauté the garlic and onions until aromatic.

Chili powder, cumin, turmeric, and curry powder should be added. For 1-2 minutes, cook.

Sweet potatoes, lentils, diced tomatoes, and vegetable broth should all be stirred in.

When the sweet potatoes are cooked and the lentils are soft, bring the mixture to a boil, then lower the heat, cover it, and simmer for 20 to 25 minutes.

To taste, add salt and pepper to the food.

Value nutritive (per serving):

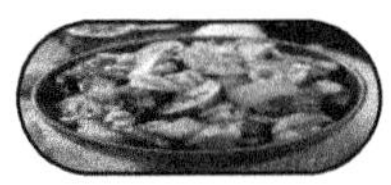

- 350 calories
- 15g of protein
- 12g of fiber
- 200mcg Folate

Preparation Time: 40–45 minutes

A parfait with berries and Greek yogurt

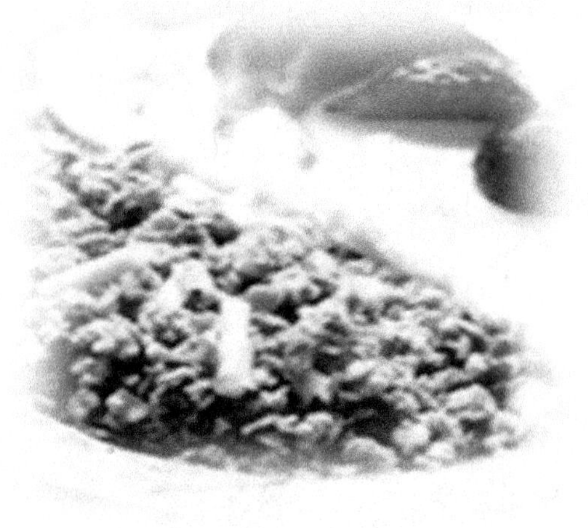

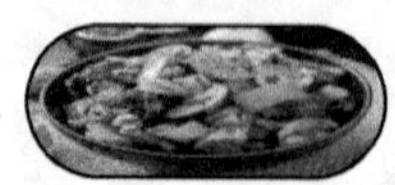

INGREDIENTS:

- Greek yogurt, one cup
- Half a cup of the mixed berries consist of strawberries, blueberries, and raspberries..
- Honey, 2 tablespoons
- Granola, 1/4 cup

PREPARATION:

- Greek yogurt, granola, and mixed berries should be arranged in a glass or bowl.
- Honey should be drizzled on top.
- If desired, repeat the layering.
- Offer cold.

VALUE NUTRITIVE (PER SERVING):

- 280 calories
- 15g of protein
- 4g of fiber
- 20mcg Folate

Preparation Time: 5 minutes–

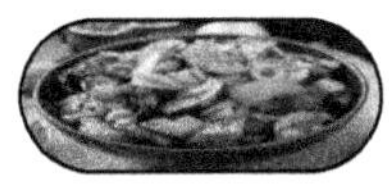

Wrap with avocado and chickpeas

INGREDIENTS:

- 1 avocado, cut into slices
- One cup of mashed chickpeas from a can
- 2 tortillas made of whole wheat
- a quarter cup of red bell pepper dice
- Red onion dice in a quarter cup
- Greek yogurt, two teaspoons
- Lemon juice, 1 tablespoon
- pepper and salt as desired

PREPARATION:

Greek yogurt, diced red bell pepper, diced red onion, mashed chickpeas, salt, and pepper should all be combined in a bowl.

Place tortillas on a table, then divide the avocado slices and chickpea mixture among them.

Serve the tortillas rolled up.–

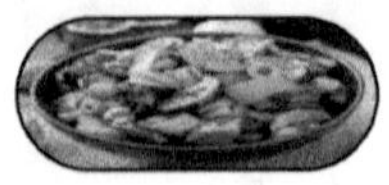

VALUE NUTRITIVE (PER SERVING):

- 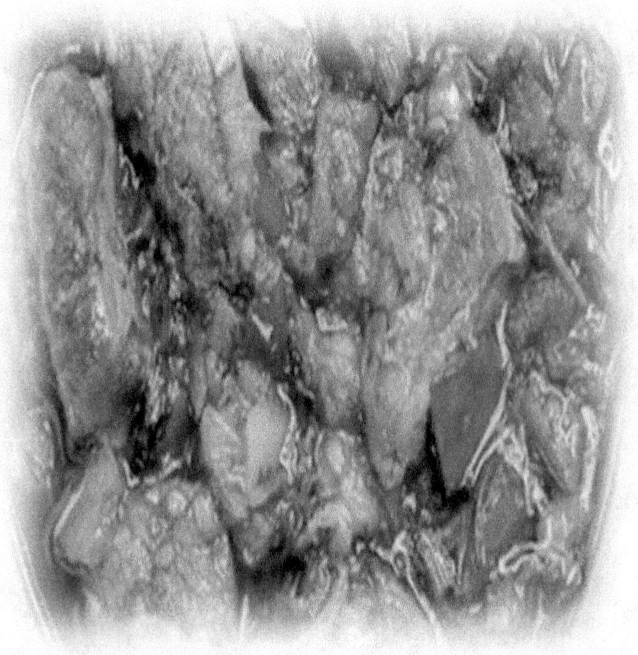 350 calories
- 10g of protein
- 10g of fiber
- 60mcg Folate

10 minutes for cooking

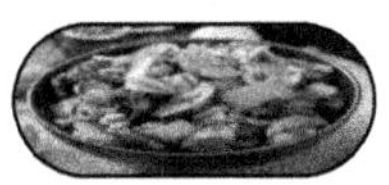

Fertility Seafood For Couples

Salmon with asparagus in a bake

INGREDIENTS:

- 2 salmon fillets, each 6 ounces
- a single asparagus bunch
- 2 minced garlic cloves
- Olive oil, 2 tablespoons
- 1 sliced lemon
- pepper and salt as desired
- garnish with fresh dill

PREPARATION:

Set your oven's temperature to 375°F (190°C).

Salmon fillets should be put on a foil-lined baking pan.

Around the fish, arrange the asparagus.

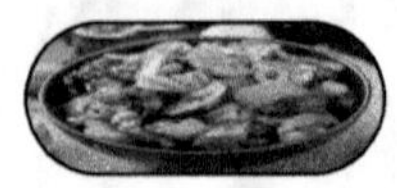

Sprinkle salt, pepper, minced garlic, and olive oil over the salmon and asparagus.

The fish should have lemon slices on it.

Bake the salmon for 15 to 20 minutes, or until it flakes easily with a fork.

Before serving, garnish with fresh dill.

VALUE NUTRITIVE (PER SERVING):

350 calories

35g of protein

1,500 mg of omega-3 fatty acids

60mcg Folate

20 minutes for cooking

Salad with shrimp and quinoa

INGREDIENTS:

- quinoa boiled to 1 cup
- Large shrimp weighing 1 pound, peeled and deveined

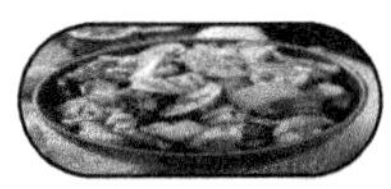

- 1 chopped red bell pepper
- Cucumber, one, diced
- 14 cup of freshly chopped parsley
- Olive oil, 2 tablespoons
- Juice of two teaspoons of lemon
- Oregano, dry, 1 teaspoon
- To taste, add salt and pepper to the dish.

PREPARATION

Cooked quinoa, diced red bell pepper, diced cucumber, and chopped parsley should all be combined in a big bowl.

Mix the olive oil, lemon juice, dried oregano, salt, and pepper in a another bowl.

For 2-3 minutes on each side, until pink and opaque, cook shrimp in a little olive oil on a skillet.

Add the cooked shrimp and the dressing to the quinoa mixture.

Serve after tossing to mix.–

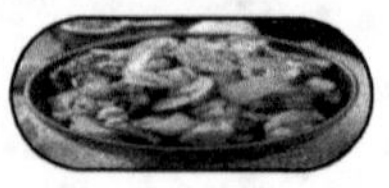

VALUE NUTRITIVE (PER SERVING):–

- 350 calories
- 30g of protein
- 5g of fiber
- 40mcg Folate

30 minutes for cooking

Salad of tuna and white beans

INGREDIENTS:

- 2 cans of drained tuna in water, each measuring 5 ounces
- 1 can (15 oz) of rinsed and drained white beans
- Red onion dice in a quarter cup
- 1/4 cup of freshly chopped basil
- Olive oil, 2 tablespoons
- Red wine vinegar, 2 teaspoons
- To taste, add salt and pepper to the dish.

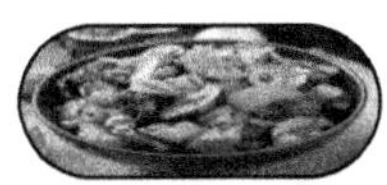

PREPARATION

Drained tuna, white beans, diced red onion, and chopped basil should all be combined in a big bowl.

Mix the olive oil, red wine vinegar, salt, and pepper in a small bowl.

On top of the tuna and bean combination, drizzle the dressing.

Before serving, toss to mix and chill.

VALUE NUTRITIVE (PER SERVING):

320 calories

30g of protein

10g of fiber

80mcg Folate

15 minutes for cooking–

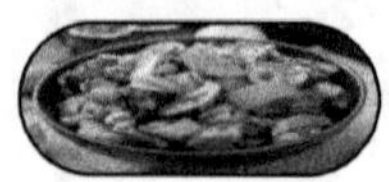

Halibut with mango salsa on the grill

INGREDIENTS:

- Two 6 oz. halibut fillets each
- One mango, diced
- A half of a red onion, finely chopped
- 1 chopped red bell pepper
- 1/4 cup freshly chopped cilantro
- Lime juice, 2 tablespoons
- Olive oil, 1 tbsp
- pepper and salt as desired

PREPARATION:

your grill temperature should be moderate in settings.

Halibut fillets should be seasoned with salt, pepper, and olive oil.

Halibut should be grilled for 3–4 minutes on each side or until it flakes easily.

Mango dice, red onion and bell pepper dice, cilantro, lime juice, and a dash of salt should all be combined in a bowl.

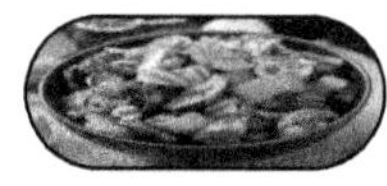

Halibut should be served grilled with mango salsa on top.

VALUE NUTRITIVE (PER SERVING):

- 320 calories
- 35g of protein
- 60 mg of vitamin C
- 40mcg Folate

10 minutes for cooking

Pasta with Lemon-Garlic Shrimp

INGREDIENTS:

- Whole wheat pasta in 8 oz.
- Large shrimp weighing 1 pound, peeled and deveined
- 3 minced garlic cloves
- 1 lemon, juiced and zesting
- Olive oil, 2 tablespoons
- 14 cup of freshly chopped parsley
- pepper and salt as desired
- Parmesan cheese, grated (optional)

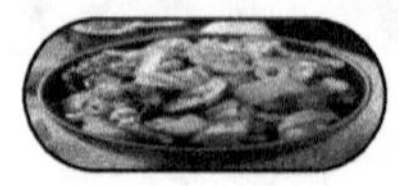

PREPARATION:

- Drain pasta after cooking it according the directions on the package.
- Olive oil should be heated to a medium-high haze in a big skillet. One minute after adding the minced garlic.
- Cook the shrimp in the skillet for two to three minutes on each side, or until pink.
- Add chopped parsley, lemon juice, and lemon zest to the skillet. Add salt and pepper to taste.
- Add the cooked pasta, shrimp, and lemon-garlic sauce to the skillet.
- Nice grated Parmesan cheese can be used in garnishing if you want to,

VALUE NUTRITIVE (PER SERVING):

- 400 calories
- 30g of protein
- 6g of fiber
- 60mcg Folate

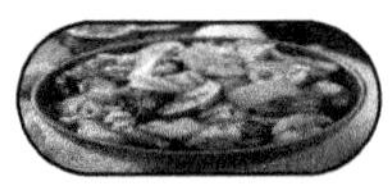

Preparation Time: 25 minutes

These seafood dishes are not only mouthwatering, but they are also packed with nutrients that can help a diet that focuses on fertility. Have fun eating!

Fertility Poultry Recipes

Grilled chicken with lemon and herbs

INGREDIENTS:

- 4 skinless, boneless breasts of chicken
- Olive oil, two tablespoons
- 2 minced garlic cloves
- 1 lemon, juiced and zesting
- Oregano, dry, 1 teaspoon
- pepper and salt as desired

—

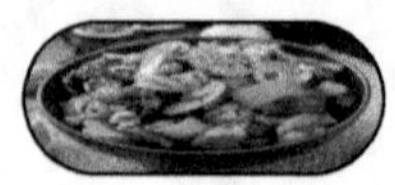

NUTRITIVE WORTH:

This dish is loaded with protein and vitamin C from the lemon, which can improve how well iron is absorbed.

PREPARATION:

- Olive oil, garlic, lemon juice, zest, oregano, salt, and pepper should all be combined in a bowl.
- Chicken breasts should be marinated in this marinade for 30 minutes.
- Heat the grill to medium-high.
- Grill chicken for 6 to 8 minutes on each side, or until done.
- To add more nutrition, serve with a side of steaming vegetables.

15-20 minutes for cooking

—

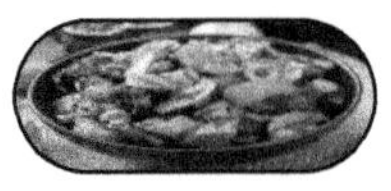

Chicken Breast Stuffed with Spinach and Tomato

INGREDIENTS:

- 4 skinless, boneless breasts of chicken
- fresh spinach greens, 2 cups
- 1 cup halved cherry tomatoes
- 1/2 cup crumbled feta cheese
- Olive oil, 1 tbsp

pepper and salt as desired

Nutritional Value: The spinach and tomatoes in this recipe contain calcium, iron, and folate.

PREPARATION:

Oven should be heated to 375°F (190°C).

Indent each chicken breast with a pocket.

Put spinach, cherry tomatoes, and feta cheese inside each breast.–

 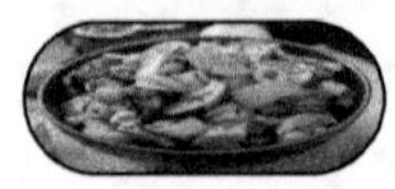

Olive oil should be drizzled over the chicken before adding salt and pepper.

Bake the chicken for 25 to 30 minutes, or until it is done.

25 to 30 minutes for cooking

Chicken with Quinoa and Veggie Stuffing

INGREDIENTS:

- 4 skinless, boneless breasts of chicken
- 1 cup cooked quinoa
- 1 cup of chopped mixed veggies, including carrots, broccoli, and bell peppers; 2 tablespoons of olive oil
- 1 paprika teaspoon
- pepper and salt as desired

Nutritional value: This recipe provides a healthy balance of chicken protein, quinoa, and vegetable fiber.

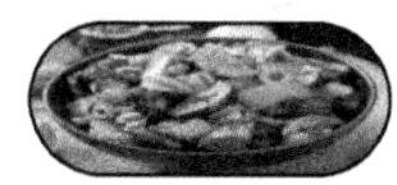

PREPARATION:

- Oven should be heated to 375°F (190°C).

- Cooked quinoa, mixed vegetables, olive oil, paprika, salt, and pepper should all be combined in a bowl.

- Each chicken breast should have a pocket created for the quinoa-vegetable mixture to be placed inside.

- Bake the chicken for 25 to 30 minutes, or until it is done.

- 25 to 30 minutes for cooking

Roasted Chicken Thighs with Lemon and Garlic

INGREDIENTS:

4 skinless, bone-in chicken thighs

zest and juice from two lemons

4 minced garlic cloves

Olive oil, two tablespoons

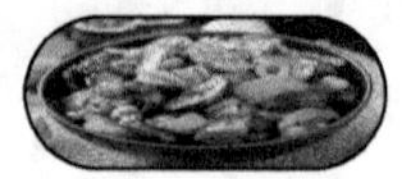

one tablespoon of dried thyme

pepper and salt as desired

Nutritional Value: The protein and vitamin C from the lemons in this recipe are both good sources.

PREPARATION:

- Oven should be heated to 400°F (200°C).
- Lemon juice, lemon zest, minced garlic, olive oil, thyme, salt, and pepper should all be combined in a bowl.
- Put this mixture on the chicken thighs.
- Roast the chicken for 25 to 30 minutes, or until it is cooked through and golden.

25 to 30 minutes for cooking

—

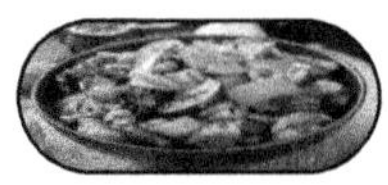

Chicken Mango Salsa

INGREDIENTS:

4 skinless, boneless breasts of chicken

One ripe mango, diced; one red bell pepper, diced; half a red onion, finely chopped; one lime, juiced; and 1/4 cup fresh cilantro, chopped

pepper and salt as desired

NUTRITIONAL VALUE: The mango, red bell pepper, and cilantro in this recipe are sources of vitamin C, folate, and antioxidants.

PREPARATION:

Chicken breasts should be salted and peppered before being grilled or fried until fully done.

To create the salsa, mix the chopped mango with the red onion, red bell pepper, cilantro, and lime juice in a basin.–

 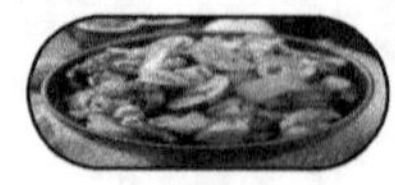

Serve the mango salsa on top of the cooked chicken.

Cooking time for chicken is 15 to 20 minutes.

These dishes can add flavor and nutrition to a diet intended to increase fertility by offering vital nutrients and well-balanced meals. Enjoy!

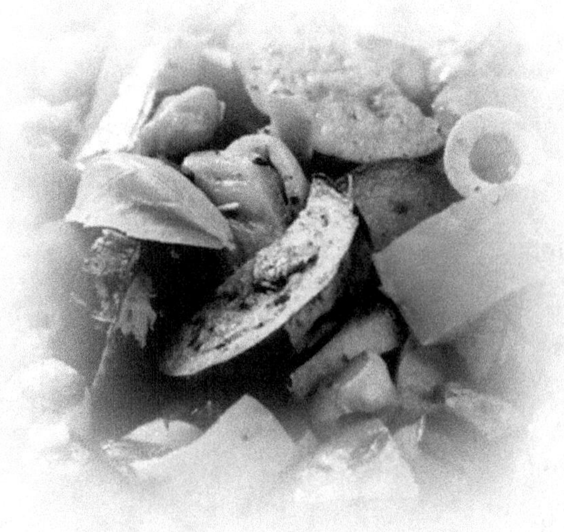

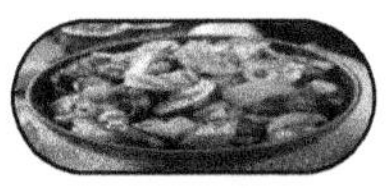

CONCLUSION

"Embark on a journey towards improved fertility with our comprehensive fertility diet cookbook designed for couples. Packed with nutrient-rich recipes and tailored meal plans, this cookbook aims to optimize fertility by promoting hormonal balance, enhancing reproductive health, and increasing the chances of conception. By incorporating wholesome foods rich in essential vitamins, minerals, and antioxidants, couples can support their fertility goals while enjoying delicious, nourishing meals. Embrace this cookbook as a holistic approach to enhance fertility and foster overall well-being.

 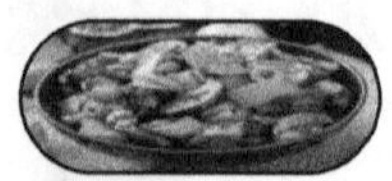

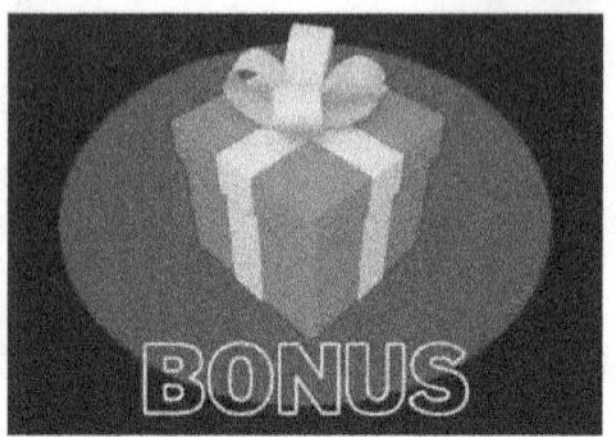

SCAN THE QR CODE TO GET YOUR FREE HOME MADE GREEN SMOOTHIE RECIPE BOOK

Your 20 days meal planner is attached at the end of the book. Enjoy!

20+ MEAL PLAN JOURNAL

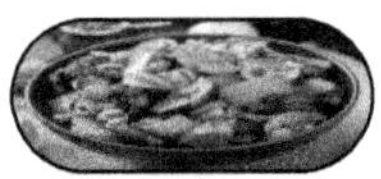

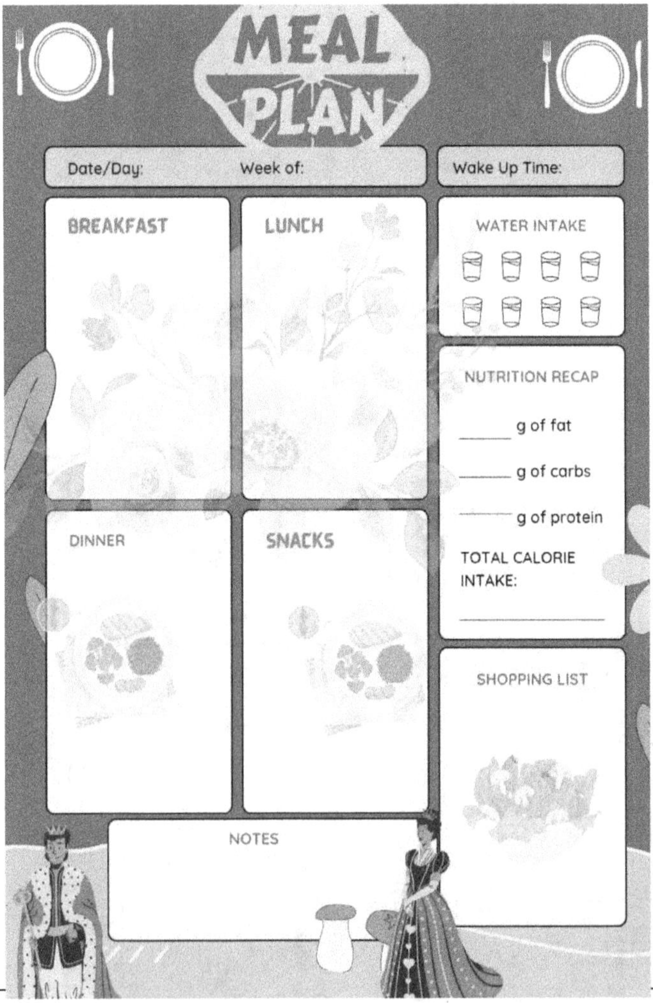

MEAL PLAN

| Date/Day: | Week of: | Wake Up Time: |

BREAKFAST

LUNCH

WATER INTAKE

NUTRITION RECAP

_______ g of fat

_______ g of carbs

_______ g of protein

TOTAL CALORIE INTAKE:

____

DINNER

SNACKS

SHOPPING LIST

NOTES

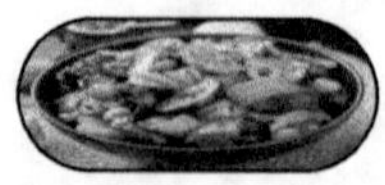

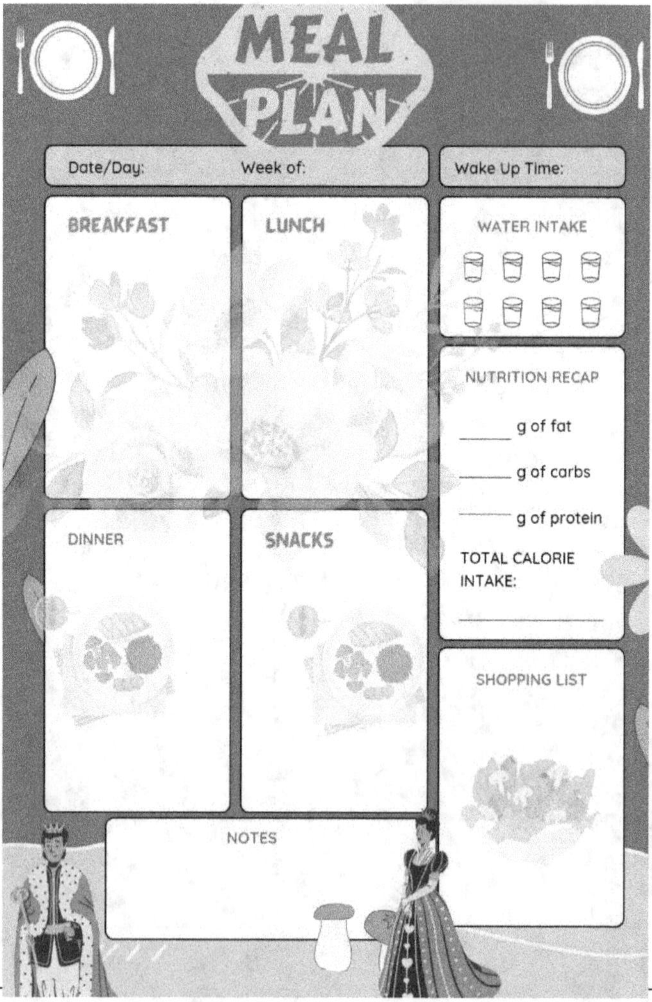

MEAL PLAN

Date/Day: Week of: Wake Up Time:

BREAKFAST

LUNCH

WATER INTAKE

NUTRITION RECAP

_______ g of fat

_______ g of carbs

_______ g of protein

TOTAL CALORIE INTAKE:

____

DINNER

SNACKS

SHOPPING LIST

NOTES

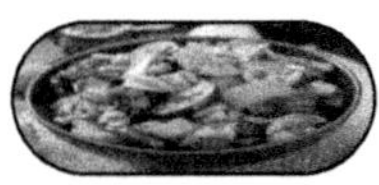

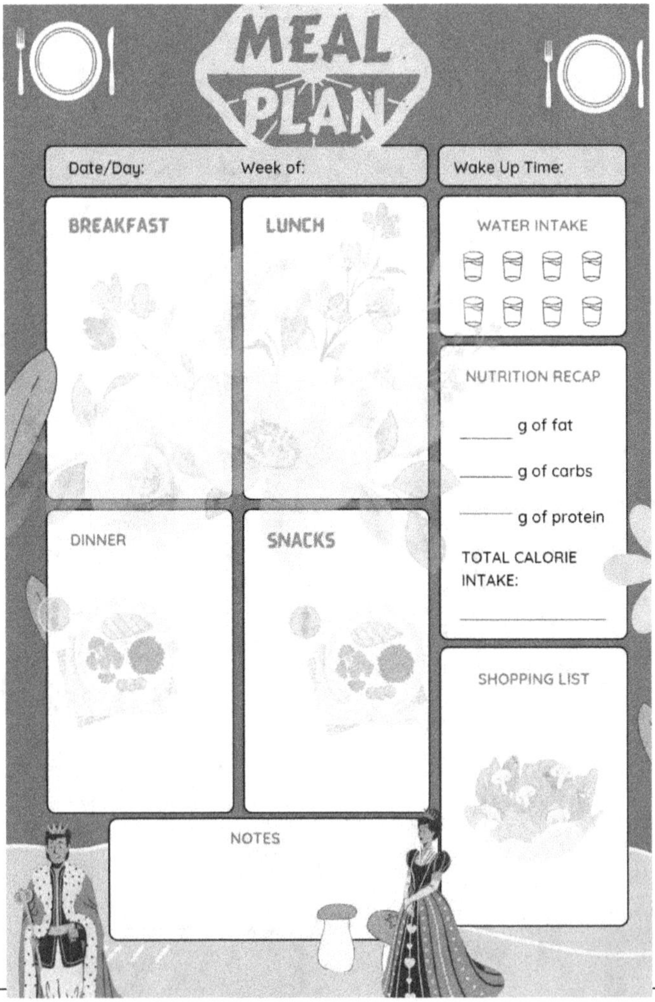

MEAL PLAN

| Date/Day: | Week of: | Wake Up Time: |

BREAKFAST

LUNCH

WATER INTAKE

NUTRITION RECAP

_______ g of fat

_______ g of carbs

_______ g of protein

TOTAL CALORIE INTAKE:

____

DINNER

SNACKS

SHOPPING LIST

NOTES

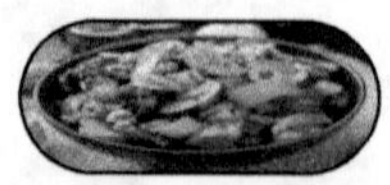

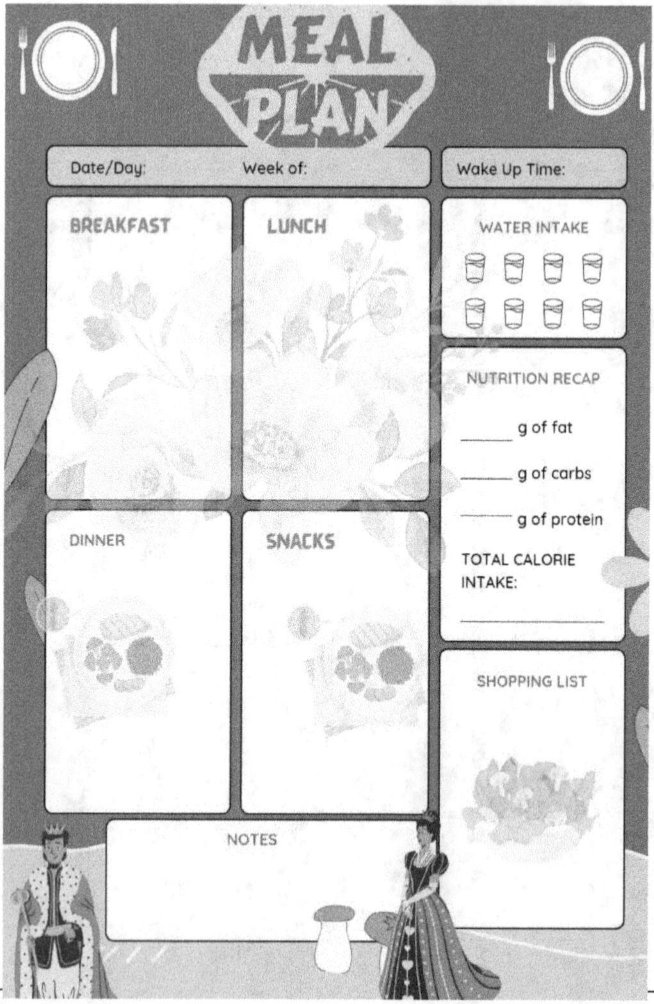

MEAL PLAN

| Date/Day: | Week of: | Wake Up Time: |

BREAKFAST

LUNCH

WATER INTAKE

NUTRITION RECAP

__________ g of fat

__________ g of carbs

__________ g of protein

TOTAL CALORIE INTAKE:

____

DINNER

SNACKS

SHOPPING LIST

NOTES

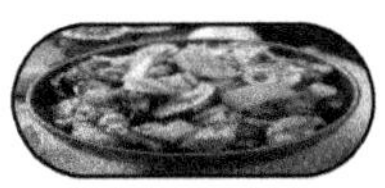

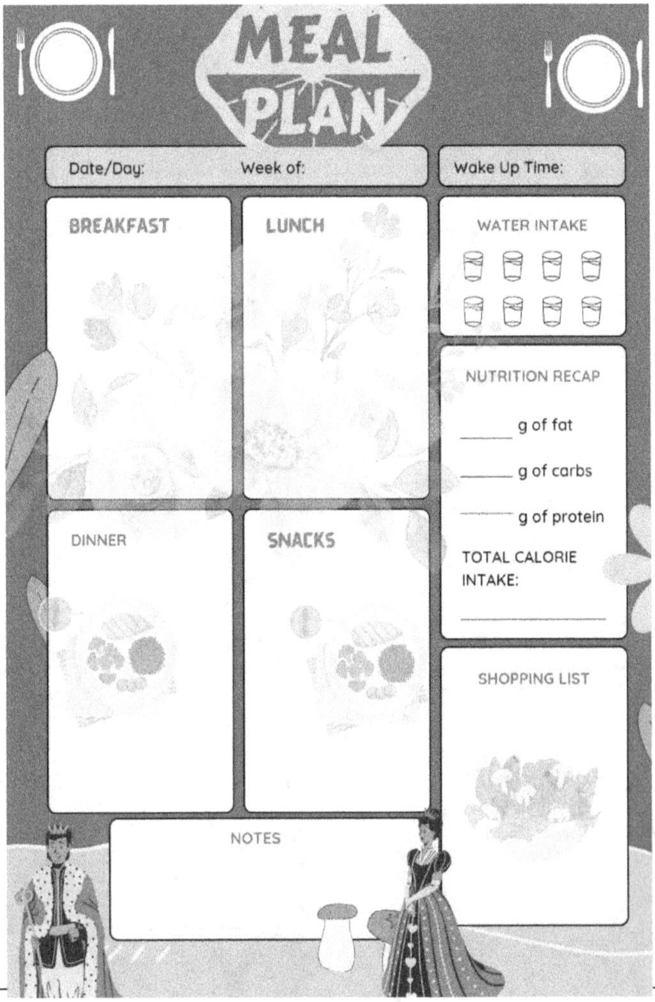

MEAL PLAN

| Date/Day: | Week of: | Wake Up Time: |

BREAKFAST

LUNCH

WATER INTAKE

NUTRITION RECAP

_______ g of fat

_______ g of carbs

_______ g of protein

TOTAL CALORIE INTAKE:

____

DINNER

SNACKS

SHOPPING LIST

NOTES

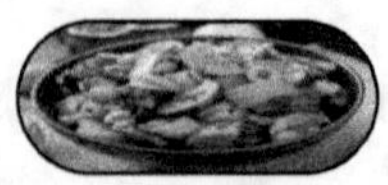

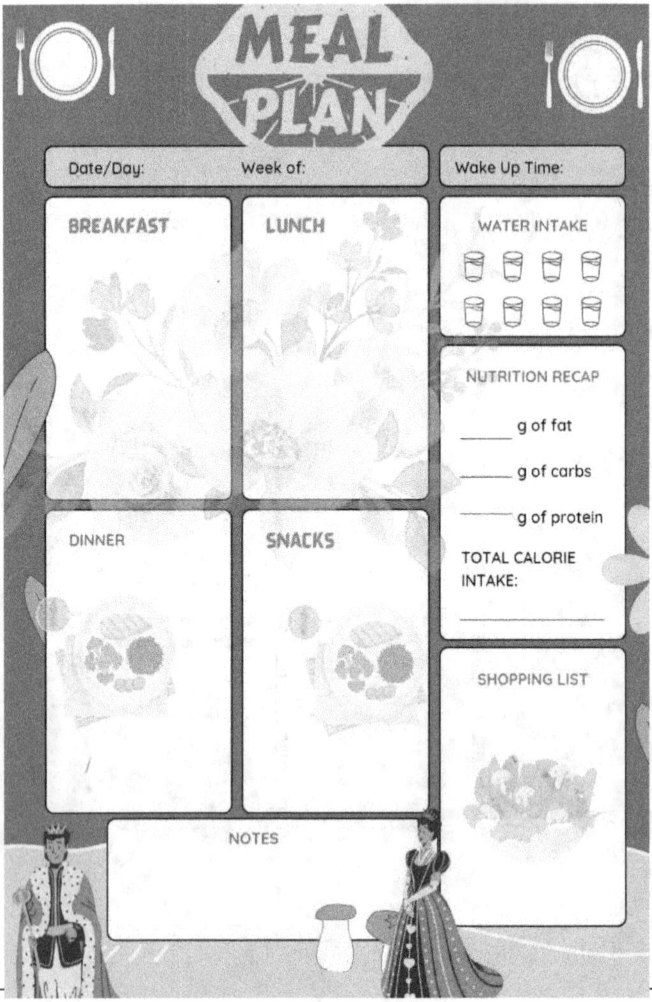

MEAL PLAN

| Date/Day: | Week of: | Wake Up Time: |

BREAKFAST

LUNCH

WATER INTAKE

NUTRITION RECAP

________ g of fat

________ g of carbs

________ g of protein

TOTAL CALORIE INTAKE:

____

DINNER

SNACKS

SHOPPING LIST

NOTES

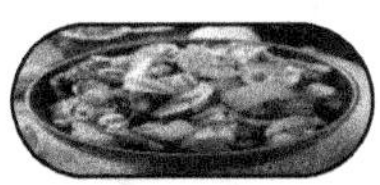

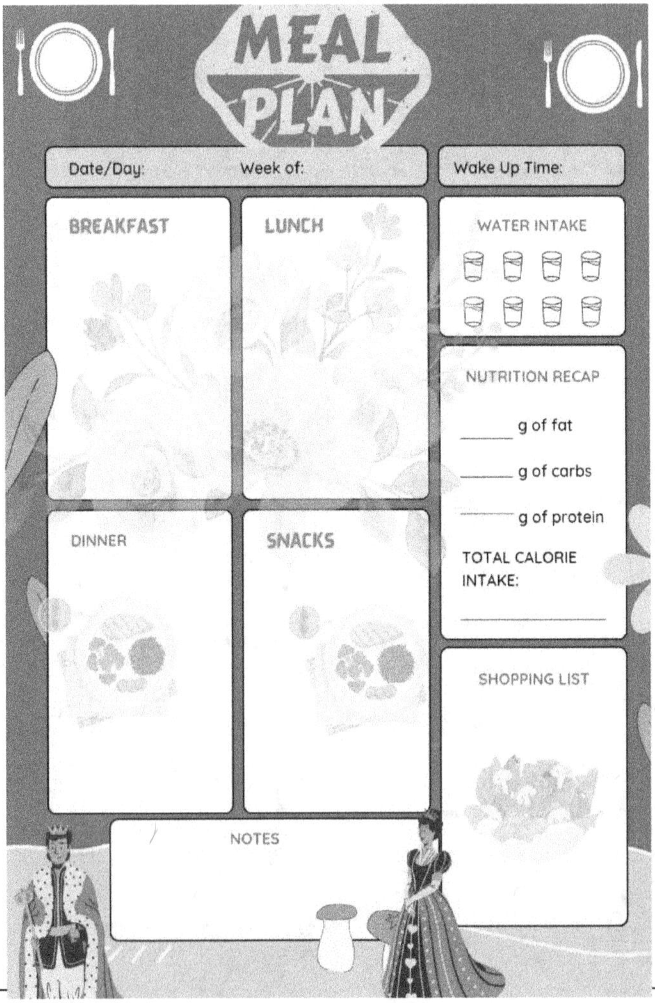

MEAL PLAN

| Date/Day: | Week of: | Wake Up Time: |

BREAKFAST

LUNCH

WATER INTAKE

NUTRITION RECAP

__________ g of fat

__________ g of carbs

__________ g of protein

TOTAL CALORIE
INTAKE:

____

DINNER

SNACKS

SHOPPING LIST

NOTES

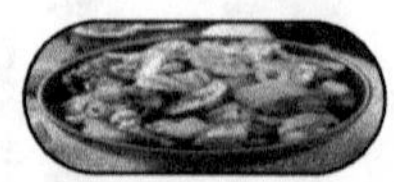

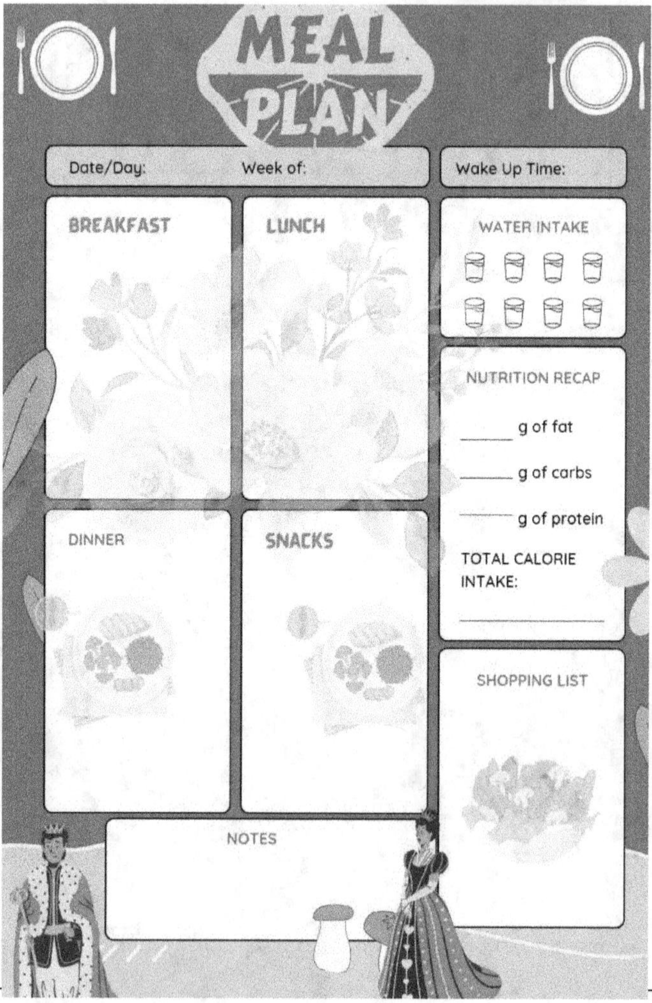

MEAL PLAN

| Date/Day: | Week of: | Wake Up Time: |

BREAKFAST

LUNCH

WATER INTAKE

NUTRITION RECAP

_______ g of fat

_______ g of carbs

_______ g of protein

TOTAL CALORIE
INTAKE:

____

DINNER

SNACKS

SHOPPING LIST

NOTES

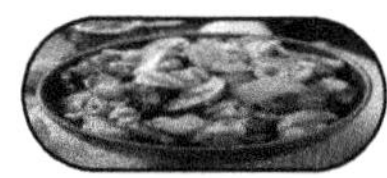

www.ingramcontent.com/pod-product-compliance
Lightning Source LLC
Chambersburg PA
CBHW060959260726
48661CB00005B/1949